SARCOIDOSIS

Discovering Sarcoidosis: Acquiring New Knowledge, Efficient Treatments, and Approaches to Respiratory Care Centered on the Patient

CHAD BRUNO

Table of Contents

Introductory

Sarcoidosis is an uncommon inflammatory illness that primarily affects the lungs and lymph nodes; however it can manifest itself in other organs as well. It is unclear what triggers sarcoidosis, however an aberrant immunological response is thought to be a contributing factor. Sarcoidosis is a condition characterized by the formation of granulomas, which are collections of inflammatory cells, anywhere in the body. These granulomas can cause inflammation and damage to the organs they form in.

• The lungs, skin, eyes, heart, liver, spleen, and nervous system are only some of the organs that sarcoidosis can impact. The severity of the disease and its symptoms vary greatly from organ to organ. A chronic cough, difficulty breathing, weakness, skin rash, joint discomfort, and vision issues are all possible symptoms.

• The diagnosis of sarcoidosis is often made after a thorough patient history is taken, a thorough physical examination is performed, diagnostic imaging procedures (such as X-rays or CT scans) are performed, and a biopsy of the afflicted tissue is taken. Mild cases of sarcoidosis may not require treatment because the illness might resolve on its own. Doctors may administer corticosteroids or other immunosuppressive drugs to minimize inflammation and control symptoms in more severe cases or when important organs are impacted.

Sarcoidosis is a disorder that requires close medical supervision and management due of its complexity and unpredictability. Patients with sarcoidosis should collaborate closely with their healthcare providers to create a tailored treatment strategy.

CHAPTER ONE
What are the Roots of Sarcoid?

Sarcoidosis has a mysterious origin that has been the focus of persistent investigation. However, there are a number of hypotheses concerning causes and factors:

- The aberrant reaction of the immune system is largely regarded to be the cause of sarcoidosis. Granulomas (small aggregates of inflammatory cells) can grow in several organs after an incorrect immune system response to an initial trigger, like exposure to an environmental or viral toxin. Still unknown is the actual antigen or trigger that sets off this immunological reaction.

• Evidence suggests that hereditary factors contribute to sarcoidosis development. It appears to be more common in particular populations and may have a hereditary propensity. Several studies have pinpointed potential causal genes for the disease.

• Exposure to particular dusts, chemicals, or diseases has been suggested as a possible environmental cause for sarcoidosis. Exposure to microbes like mycobacteria has been studied as a possible cause, however the results have been unconvincing.

- Occupational exposures: a subtype of sarcoidosis, berylliosis, has been linked to the metal beryllium, which some people may have been exposed to in the course of their work.

Although they are hypothesized to play a role in triggering or exacerbating sarcoidosis, the illness is likely impacted by a combination of genetic and environmental factors, and its precise origin remains unknown. The symptoms and severity of sarcoidosis vary greatly from person to person and between age groups and cultural groups. Scientists are still trying to figure out what causes this illness so that they can come up with better ways to treat it.

Definitions and Classifications of Sarcoidosis

Because of its wide-ranging effects, sarcoidosis is often categorized according to the affected organs and the severity of the disease. Sarcoidosis can be characterized by its progression and severity according to its type and stage. The Scadding staging system is the gold standard for sarcoidosis categorization, and it divides the illness into five stages:

• Stage 0: At this point, the damaged organs show no granulomas or other symptoms of active illness. No granulomas are evident, however sarcoidosis may be suspected due to symptoms or other diagnostic findings.

• Lymph nodes, especially those in the chest (hilar and mediastinal lymph nodes), include granulomas at this stage.

• Second-stage disease is characterized by the presence of granulomas in additional sites outside the lymph nodes, most frequently the lungs. Two additional categories make up Stage II:

Stage II A: Lymph nodes are the only site where granulomas have spread to.

Granulomas are found in the lymph nodes and the afflicted organ(s) at Stage II B.

• Granulomas are present in the site(s) of organ involvement but not in the lymph nodes at this stage. It's possible for the disease to manifest in other organs besides the skin, eyes, liver, and spleen.

- Stage IV sarcoidosis is the most advanced form of the disease and is characterized by widespread fibrosis (scarring) throughout the organs affected. This stage can lead to serious organ malfunction and damage.

It's worth noting that not all sarcoidosis cases move through all these stages, and that some people may stay in one stage for a very long period or forever. Sarcoidosis, especially in its milder types, can sometimes go into remission or resolve on its own.

Sarcoidosis is classified not only by the stages it progresses through but also by the organs it affects. Depending on the affected organ(s), sarcoidosis can manifest in a number of different ways.

• When the lungs are the primary site of involvement, the condition is called pulmonary sarcoidosis. This is the most typical manifestation of the illness.

• Skin lesions, rashes, or nodules are typical of the cutaneous form of sarcoidosis.

• Ocular sarcoidosis: When sarcoidosis spreads to the eyes, it can cause inflammation, dryness, and impaired vision.

• Neurosarcoidosis is characterized by a wide variety of neurological symptoms caused by damage to the central nervous system (brain and spinal cord).

• Sarcoidosis of the heart, often called cardiac sarcoidosis, is a serious condition that can cause arrhythmias, heart failure, and other cardiovascular complications.

Symptoms, available treatments, and overall prognosis for sarcoidosis patients are all affected by the disease's kind and stage. The diagnosis and treatment of sarcoidosis require the expertise of a medical practitioner.

CHAPTER TWO
Alternative Treatments

Sarcoidosis treatment varies from patient to patient based on disease severity, affected organs, and symptoms. In the event of moderate forms of the disease that do not severely impair organ function, treatment may be unnecessary. However, when treatment is necessary, it typically targets inflammation reduction, symptom management, and complication prevention or treatment. Sarcoidosis typically responds well to the following treatments:

- In many cases, the initial treatment for sarcoidosis is corticosteroids like prednisone. They aid in decreasing inflammation and tamping down on the immune system's overreaction. Treatment with corticosteroids may last for a shorter or longer period of time depending on the severity of the condition and the patient's response. In some circumstances, long-term use is required, however because of the risk of adverse effects, it is imperative that patients be closely monitored.

- Medication to inhibit the immune system and regulate inflammation, such as methotrexate, azathioprine, or mycophenolate mofetil, may be recommended to patients who do not react to or who cannot tolerate corticosteroids.

• Treatment with biologic medicines such as infliximab, adalimumab, or rituximab may be considered for patients with severe or resistant sarcoidosis. When conventional treatments have failed, these medications may be tried because they focus on specific pathways within the immune system.

• Topical corticosteroids or other topical therapies may be used to control skin problems in patients with sarcoidosis.

• Pulmonary sarcoidosis patients can benefit from exercise, education, and social support offered by pulmonary rehabilitation centers.

• Medications and treatments may be administered to alleviate some symptoms and consequences associated with sarcoidosis. Joint pain can be treated with nonsteroidal anti-inflammatory medicines (NSAIDs), while ocular sarcoidosis is treated with eye drops.

• Regular checkups and monitoring are necessary to track the development of the condition, make any necessary adjustments to treatment, and deal with any unwanted drug effects.

• Surgery: When alternative therapies fail or when organs are severely affected, surgery may be essential to remove granulomas or resolve consequences.

Patients with sarcoidosis must collaborate closely with doctors who are familiar with the disease. The specifics of each patient's treatment plan should be determined as the condition progresses. Some patients with sarcoidosis may go into remission on their own, while others may continue to endure symptoms indefinitely. In order to keep the disease under control and improve the patient's quality of life, consistent medical checkups are needed.

Medical therapy, behavioral modifications, and close monitoring are all part of the management of sarcoidosis. Key measures for optimal sarcoidosis management include:

1. The intricate nature of sarcoidosis necessitates the

involvement of healthcare specialists with expertise in managing the ailment. Your care may involve a rheumatologist, a pulmonologist, or another expert, depending on which organs are affected.

2. Follow Your Treatment Plan: If your healthcare practitioner recommends medicine, take it as instructed. Know what to expect and talk to your doctor right away if you experience any adverse reactions.

3. Due to the unpredictability of sarcoidosis, constant monitoring is essential. Your doctor will examine you, determine whether or not any treatment changes are necessary, and keep an eye out for any adverse effects.

4. Modifications to Your Way of Life The following modifications to your way of life may aid in the management of sarcoidosis:

Smoking can exacerbate lung involvement in sarcoidosis, therefore if you smoke, you should try to quit.

• **Maintain a Healthy Diet:** Eating a balanced and healthy diet can assist your overall health. Talk to your doctor or a certified dietitian if your sarcoidosis has caused you to have dietary limits or worries.

Regular exercise is important for maintaining healthy lungs and a healthy body. Exercise can help you feel better, but it's important to talk to your doctor before starting any new routine.

• **De-stress:** Living with a chronic illness like sarcoidosis can be trying. Think about trying some meditation, mindfulness, or relaxation techniques to calm your nerves.

5. Connecting with individuals who have sarcoidosis or joining a support group can be a great source of moral support and knowledge. Participating in such forums might teach you how other people have handled similar situations.

6. Protect against Infections: Since sarcoidosis involves an aberrant immune response, it's vital to take precautions against infections. Avoiding close contact with sick people is an important part of infection prevention, as is using proper hand hygiene and having the appropriate vaccines.

7. If you have cutaneous or ocular sarcoidosis, it's important to avoid direct sunlight and other irritants to avoid aggravating your skin and eyes. Protect your eyes with sunglasses and sunscreen.

8. Medications for sarcoidosis should be taken regularly and exactly as prescribed. Consult your doctor if you have any uncomfortable symptoms.

9. Sarcoidosis can go into remission and then flare up, so it's important to be prepared for both. You and your doctor should formulate a strategy for dealing with worsening symptoms in the event that they occur.

10. Get the facts about sarcoidosis from reliable sources. Find out what's wrong, what could go wrong, and what treatments are out there. You can use this information to better guide your healthcare decisions.

Keep in mind that everyone with sarcoidosis is different; therefore your treatment plan should be customized for you. Changes in your health status, responses to therapy, and your general well-being are all topics that should be discussed openly and frequently with your healthcare team.

Frequent Difficulties

Complications from sarcoidosis can vary in type and severity depending on the damaged organ and the disease's progression in a given individual. The following are examples of typical sarcoidosis complications:

• Scarring of lung tissue, known as pulmonary fibrosis, can reduce lung capacity.

Pulmonary hypertension is a condition in which the heart has to work more than usual to pump blood around the body.

Common symptoms like chronic cough and shortness of breath can have a major influence on quality of life.

• **Eye problems:** Sarcoidosis can damage the eyes, leading to problems like uveitis (inflammation of the uvea), conjunctivitis (inflammation of the conjunctiva), and potentially visual impairment.

• Symptoms of cutaneous sarcoidosis include the development of lesions, nodules, and scarring on the skin, which can be both painful and unsightly.

- Complications involving the heart include arrhythmias, heart block, and even heart failure caused by cardiac sarcoidosis.

- Headaches, eye issues, seizures, and mental abnormalities are just some of the neurological complications that can arise from neurosarcoidosis, which is an inflammation of the central nervous system.

- Complications with the kidneys (renal) are uncommon with sarcoidosis, but might include kidney stones, reduced kidney function, and even kidney failure.

- Complications of the Musculoskeletal System Joint pain and swelling, similar to the symptoms of arthritis, can occur in some circumstances.

- Hepatomegaly (liver enlargement) and higher liver enzyme levels are two possible outcomes of sarcoidosis's impact on the liver.

- Abdominal pain, diarrhea, and other digestive disorders are possible complications of gastrointestinal tract involvement.

- Hypercalcemia: Sarcoidosis can cause the body to create too much calcium, which can lead to a range of symptoms, including kidney stones, bone pain, and weariness.

• The risk of secondary infections is elevated when immunosuppressive drugs are used to treat sarcoidosis. If a patient notices any of these symptoms, they should seek medical attention immediately.

It's worth noting that not everyone with sarcoidosis will have these symptoms, and some people may have a minor case that resolves on its own. The diagnosis and therapy of sarcoidosis are generally adjusted to the individual problems and organ involvement in each patient. Constant check-ups by medical staff are necessary for early detection of problems and appropriate response.

Conclusion

Sarcoidosis is a multi-organ inflammatory illness that can manifest in a number of different ways from one patient to the next. The specific cause of sarcoidosis is unknown, however it is thought to be related to a malfunctioning immune system, which could be driven by both hereditary and environmental causes. Sarcoidosis treatment is a team effort that calls for input from a wide range of medical specialists.

• Different sarcoidosis treatments are available depending on the severity of the disease, the afflicted organs, and the patient's symptoms. Corticosteroids, immunosuppressive drugs, and, in extreme situations, biologic medicines are frequently used as therapy modalities. Modifications to one's way of life, consistent monitoring, and a strong support system can all play significant roles in the control of the disease.

• The severity of consequences from sarcoidosis is proportional to the number of organs that are affected. Lungs, eyes, skin, the heart, the neurological system, and other organs and systems could be impacted by these issues. A patient's quality of life can be improved by preventative care, including regular checkups and open conversation with their healthcare providers about any concerns they may have.

Although sarcoidosis is difficult to control, many people are able to do so with the help of medical treatment and by taking preventative measures. Researchers hope that by learning more about what causes sarcoidosis and how to cure it, they can help those who suffer from it.

THE END